Juicing and weight loss: a comprehensive guide to juice recipes and weight loss juicing.

Thomas J. Schmidt

Table of contents

Chapter 1.

The basics of juicing and blending.

Juicing and Blending Basics
From using a juicer to picking the best ingredients, here's the everything guide to fresh fruit and vegetable drinks.
For the juice obsessed, the smoothie fanatic, the blender beginner, or the juicing novice, here's how to enhance your experience and get the most out of both your appliances and your ingredients. Because whether you've resolved to break out your blender or break out of your rut, know that there are two trends that have withstood the test of time: trying new things and eating your veggies.

Juicers

There are two kinds of juicers: masticating and centrifugal. Masticating juicers, which are a little slower, "chew" the product to separate solid from liquid, which is moderately more efficient at getting every last drop of juice out. Centrifugal models spin the fruit and vegetables around to separate the juice from the pulp, which is faster than masticating.

Blenders

As far as blenders go, there are high-performance blenders and regular blenders.

High-performance machines let you incorporate harder products such as nuts easily. They also puree foods at incredibly high speeds, and they may even have pre-programmed settings for super-efficient blending.

Regular blenders tend to be much more affordable and a bit less powerful than high-performance machines — many are daunted by ice or nuts — so if you have one, use the tricks below to make blending a breeze.

Shoot for seasonal and organic whenever possible: Almost everything tastes better both local and in season. If you can afford organic, go for it, especially for delicate berries or anything without a skin that you discard.

Wash your produce: Thoroughly wash your produce (even if it's organic). Since you're not cooking or pasteurizing the juice, it's a handy way to reduce bacteria.

The myth about pith: When juicing citrus, peel the fruits well, but leave behind a little white pith. It can be mildly bitter, but it also contains pectin and bioflavonoids, which help the body absorb vitamin C.

Build a better smoothie: Add smoothie ingredients in a specific order so your blender operates as efficiently as possible. From first to last: harder (nuts, seeds, dried and frozen fruits), softer (nut butter, fresh fruits, and vegetables), powdered (cacao, protein, supplements), liquid (the choice is yours). Ice can be added at any time.

Get the most out of your greens: Pack leafy greens in between juicier items like apples or cucumbers to help get the most juice out of them. Or, if you have multiple speed settings, tightly pack your greens into balls that fit into the feed chute and juice them at low speed.

A tough nut to crack: Want to incorporate nuts into your smoothies but don't have a high-powered blender? Soak the nuts in water for at least 2 hours and up to a day and blend with liquid.

Sweeten your smoothies with something different: Dried fruit (like dates) is great for adding sweetness. For extra-smooth blending, soak them in water for up to 20 minutes to rehydrate them before adding them to the carafe.

Make the most of your pulp: Juicing leaves behind a lot of pulp, but it doesn't have to end up in the trash. Consider using your pulp in baked goods or soups. Carrot muffins, anyone?

Drinking
Consume drinks quickly: Fresh juices and smoothies deteriorate and oxidize with extended exposure to air, so drink them soon after you juice them.
Eat your vegetables — or drink a few: Juicing is a great way to round out your daily fruit and vegetable intake, but definitely don't forget about whole fruits and vegetables either.

Chapter 2

WaterMelon juice.

How to Make Watermelon Juice

 ingredients. You will need:
seedless watermelon
Powdered sugar or honey to taste. Cold water and ice cubes, Place your watermelon on a cutting board. Peel the watermelon and slice it into (2.5 cm) chunks using a sharp knife.
Place the watermelon chunks into a bowl, into a rubber container, or onto a plate. Use a fork instead of using your hands to prevent messiness.
Place the watermelon in a blender. Add powdered sugar or honey, if desired.
Blend your watermelon chunks and sweetener and check the consistency.
Add water for thinner juice and add ice cubes for thicker juice.
Blend well until the juice is smooth. Pour the juice over ice cubes into a tall glass. You

can strain the juice, if you wish, to remove the pulp.

Heated Lemon Watermelon Juice

Gather your ingredients. You will need:

7 sprigs of mint

Juice of 1 1/2 lemons

1 tablespoon of sugar

2 small seedless watermelons

Cut the rinds off the watermelons. Slice the flesh into (2.5 cm) chunks.

Blend the chunks, mint, and lemon juice until the mixture is smooth.

Pour the watermelon mixture through a sieve and into a saucepan. Press down on the watermelon using a wooden spoon to release the most juice. Mix the juice with sugar.

Heat your saucepan over a medium-low setting. Bring the juice to a simmer, but don't allow it to boil.

Continue simmering the juice. Taste it frequently to see how the flavors are developing. When the juice is ready, remove it from the heat and let it cool.

Pour the juice into a container and chill it. Serve the chilled juice in a tall glass over ice. Garnish the juice with a mint leaf.

Wash the watermelon well. Remove dirt or blemishes.

Peel a seedless watermelon.

Separate the rind from the flesh of the watermelon. Chop it up.

Put the chopped pieces of watermelon rind into the blender. Blend until it reaches the desired consistency.

Add water if needed.

Serve and enjoy!

Watermelon 7Up Juice

Gather your ingredients. The things you will need are as follows:

Half of the medium Watermelon

3 Teaspoon sugar

A pinch of salt (if you like.)

1 Glass of 7Up

1 tablespoon lemon Juice

Ice cubes

Peel the watermelon and slice it into small chunks using a knife. Put the watermelon in the juicer. Add sugar, salt, and lemon juice. Strain it into a glass

Serve it with 7Up and an office cube. How can I naturally preserve watermelon juice?

Put it in the fridge, or if you want it to be Slushie-ish, freeze it. How long can watermelon be kept in the refrigerator?

A whole watermelon can stay in the refrigerator for up to 2 weeks. Leave the white rind intact; it contains more vitamins and nutrients than the red flesh.

Always use a ripe watermelon for juicing. If you like sweetness, select a sweeter variety of watermelon, such as sugar baby. Fresh mint makes a vibrant addition to watermelon juice. Add a few clean mint leaves to the juice as it is blending.

To make blended watermelon juice, slice a watermelon into 1-inch chunks and pour them into a blender. Add cold water, ice cubes, and powdered sugar or honey for a sweeter juice. Blend until the mixture is smooth. For a fresher taste, consider adding mint and lemon juice, or mixing and matching with other fruits like raspberries and pomegranate seeds. Add 7-Up for a crisp, carbonated flavor. For a healthy juice recipe made using the watermelon's rind.

Chapter 3

Fruits

Bananas
Rich in soluble fiber, bananas are an easy grab-and-go snack that can help lower cholesterol. For an extra heart-healthy boost, slice bananas on top of morning oats with a tablespoon of chia seeds and walnuts. It's a hearty, energy-packed breakfast loaded with fiber, vitamin B6, potassium, magnesium, vitamin C, and manganese.

Oranges
You already knew that oranges came packed with vitamin C, but get this: Citrus fruits have been shown to have anti-inflammatory, antioxidative, and anti-cancer properties, according to research published in Chemistry Central Journal. Oranges are

wonderful on their own, sliced into a salad, or used in cooking or baking.

Grapes

Grapes contain polyphenolic compounds with antioxidant properties, which may help reduce cellular damage. Adding grapes (about 1–2 cups per day) to your diet can help to protect your body's tissues and decrease markers of inflammation. Frozen grapes are a wonderful, hydrating summer treat, but also consider roasting grapes along with veggies on a sheet pan!

Guava

Give your immune system a boost with guava. They're rich in vitamin C, potassium, and fiber, and have a fair amount of folate. With a tropical tang, guavas can be used to make a tasty jam or turned into a syrup or glaze to use in a host of recipes.

Cantaloupe melon slices.

Cantaloupe is high in potassium, vitamin C and folate. The flavonoids found in melon have anti-inflammatory, blood sugar-stabilizing, and immune-boosting properties. Plus, water-filled cantaloupe offers a hydration boost. You can make a cool salad with cantaloupe and cucumber, with granola sprinkled on top for a bit of crunch!

Strawberries
Strawberries are a great source of antioxidants — especially vitamin C. Just one cup of halved strawberries packs about 150% of your daily value. The same serving also contains about 80 calories and up to 9 grams of fiber, a combo that helps you enjoy maximum flavor and fullness for a minimal number of calories. Use their sweetness to create wonderful desserts!

Grapefruit
Like another citrus, grapefruit packs tons of vitamin C. Research has shown that

consuming grapefruit improves blood pressure and may help to lower cholesterol levels. Make it easy to get those citrusy sections with a grapefruit knife and add them to salad, yogurt, granola, or oatmeal.

Blackberries
Blackberries provide nature's perfect snack: They're deliciously sweet, satisfying, and nutrient-packed. One cup can provide about half of the vitamin C you need each day. Plus, they're a good source of both vitamin K and manganese. Our favorite way to eat any type of berries? Swap them for the jam to add extra fiber, more antioxidants, and less sugar.

Avocado.
Avocado is a unique fruit (yep, it's a fruit!) because of its low sugar content. It also provides heart-healthy fatty acids and magnesium, a key mineral linked to neurological and muscular function. You

know all about avocado toast, but have you tried adding avocado to your smoothies?

Plums
Plums have been shown to have anti-inflammatory benefits that may help to boost cognition. Choose dried prunes for even more calcium and magnesium, which have been linked to decreasing your risk of osteoporosis. Or when you're grilling chicken or a steak, throw on some halved fresh plums — the heat intensifies their sweetness.

Blueberry
Since they're loaded with polyphenolic compounds, eating more blueberries can protect your heart by benefiting blood vessels and deter harmful plaque or damage. The fiber in berries also slows down the rate of digestion in your GI tract, steadying the release of sugar into your bloodstream and offering a longer-lasting energy boost. Besides adding them to anything from

oatmeal and yogurt to salads and grain dishes, consider the most obvious and delicious option: blueberry muffins!

Lemons
Lemons are high in vitamin C, folate, potassium, and flavonoids. Flavonoids have been linked to reducing your risk of cognitive decline by enhancing circulation and helping to protect brain cells from damage. Lemons add brightness to so many dishes, from savory to sweet.

Raspberries
Raspberries are one of the highest-fiber fruits, with one cup containing 8 grams. As a nutrient-packed choice, raspberries provide antioxidants and blood-sugar stabilizing benefits, especially when combined with a source of protein. Add 'em to your breakfast, whether that's oatmeal, a smoothie, or yogurt — it'll help boost your energy levels and keep you satisfied until lunchtime.

Green pears

Besides vitamin C and fiber (25% of your daily value!), a single juicy pear will also help keep you hydrated. One quick dinner idea: This Thai steak and pear salad recipe from the Good Housekeeping Test Kitchen takes only 20 minutes to make. And like plums, pears are wonderful grilled as a side dish to whatever protein main dish you're BBQing.

Pomegranate

One cup of these petite treats packs up to 7 grams of filling fiber and 10% of the potassium you should get per day. They're also a decent source of both vitamin C and vitamin K. Use them in savory entrées or sprinkle them into salads for a hint of sweetness. The arils (or seeds) have a bit of a crunch, making them a nice addition to yogurt as well.

Limes
Limes have some nice health benefits: They're loaded with vitamin C and are a decent source of calcium and iron. They're great in a margarita, of course, and are terrific in Thai-inspired recipes, like this seared coconut-lime chicken dish. A good tool to have on hand to make the most of all citrus fruit is a well-made zester.

Honeydew melons
Sweet honeydews are another fruit that packs a nice punch of vitamin C: It provides over 50% of your daily value. They'll also give you a burst of potassium and fiber. Honeydew is a nice addition to a cool summery soup, like one made with cucumbers and lime juice.

Pineapple
This tropical fruit is simply loaded with vitamin C and is an excellent source of manganese, a mineral that helps your brain and nervous system function. Pineapple is

one of the best fruits to grill, whether it's for a main meal side dish or as the base for an excellent dessert.

Breadfruit
Another great source of vitamin C, breadfruit also has a fair amount of the minerals potassium and magnesium. It's particularly interesting because when it's unripe it can be cooked like a potato, but when it's ripe it can be used in a dessert. Another thing that's unusual about breadfruit: It's a terrific source of protein.

Chapter 4

Vegetables and their benefits in weight loss

The Benefits of Vegetables for Weight Loss
If your goal is to lose weight, you might want to start by re-examining what is on your plate. It can be hard to lose weight if you are not eating the right types of meals. The best type of food for weight loss is going to be whole foods that are unprocessed and preferably organic.

Vegetables are a natural weight loss food and some of the healthiest food that you can eat. They are low in calories and fat plus they are high in fiber which can help keep you fuller for longer. As a bonus, they can help you de-bloat and lower inflammation throughout your body.

Weekly vegetable amounts: You want to make sure you are eating a wide variety of vegetables so that you can soak up their nutrients such as fiber, antioxidants, vitamins, and minerals to help keep you healthy. Below are the weekly amounts and types of vegetables that you should be eating based on the USDA vegetable recommendations.

The USDA recommends that you should be eating a variety of vegetables WEEKLY from the following subgroups:

Dark-green vegetables: 1 ½ cups

Red & orange vegetables: 5 ½ cups

Beans & peas: 1 ½ cups

Starchy vegetables: 5 cups

Other vegetables: 4 cups

The amounts above are for women. Men should add about a half cup of vegetables to each of these amounts.

Daily vegetable amounts: According to the USDA vegetable guidelines for adults, you should be consuming about 2-3 cups of vegetables per day. I encourage my clients to get around 3 cups of vegetables per day. The more active you are, the more vegetables you need to include in your diet.

Nutrients you get from vegetables when you are eating a varied diet:

Fiber: Another benefit to eating vegetables is they contain fiber which helps to slow digestion, keeping you fuller longer and helping to balance blood sugar. According to the FDA, Americans should consume 28 grams of fiber per day if they're following an it2,000i calorie diet.

Antioxidants: Vegetables also contain antioxidants that can prevent or slow damage to cells caused by free radicals protecting you from certain types of cancers. Antioxidant-rich vegetables; broccoli, spinach, carrots, potatoes, artichokes, cabbage, asparagus, alfa sprouts, beets, onions, collard greens, and kale.

Vitamins and minerals: Vegetables are an important source of many nutrients that help keep you healthy by lowering your risk of chronic diseases such as heart disease, and certain types of cancers, they can help lower blood pressure, improve digestion, and have a positive effect on blood sugar.

Vitamin A: sweet potatoes, carrots, collard greens, swiss chard, spinach, kale, winter squash, red pepper

Vitamin K: broccoli, Brussel sprouts, collard greens, swiss chard, spinach, kale, mustard greens

Vitamin C: broccoli, Brussels sprouts, sweet yellow peppers, kale, mustard greens, chili peppers

Folate (folic acid): asparagus, beets, broccoli, sprouts, spinach, kale

Potassium: swiss chard, acorn squash, spinach, bok choy, mushrooms, sweet potatoes, brussel sprouts, broccoli, artichoke, green peas, asparagus

Magnesium: spinach, swiss chard, acorn squash, artichoke, green peas, kale, okra, potatoes

Iron: collard greens, swiss chard, spinach, kale, potatoes, mushrooms

Calcium: collard greens, spinach, kale, rhubarb

How to build a plate when weight loss is your goal:

When trying to lose weight, I recommend you first fill half your plate with vegetables, then focus on adding a low-fat organic protein, a portion of carbohydrates, and a small portion of healthy fat to complete your plate.

If weight loss is your goal, I recommend you eat the vegetables on your plate first. You might want to eat a salad before your main meal or you can just start with the vegetables that are on your plate. When you eat your vegetables first, you are filling up on the lowest calorie food first and it can help you feel more full throughout your meal. As you can see, there are so many more benefits of eating vegetables than just losing weight. They are an essential part of our diet to keep you healthy and strong for life.

Chapter 5

Juicing and weight loss.

Weight LossDiets
Is Juicing Good for Weight Loss? Here's What Doctors Say
It might seem like a quick way to drop pounds, but experts say it's not that simple.

Preview for 8 Practical Tips for Weight Loss
If you're trying to lose weight, juicing might sound like a slam-dunk approach guaranteed to produce quick results. After all, juice derives exclusively from whole fruits and veggies, so it must be a healthy way to get to a lean body, right? It's not quite that simple.
"We all know that getting our daily dose of fruits and vegetables is essential for overall health and well-being," explains Dr. Mahmud Kara, M.D., who previously treated patients at the Cleveland Clinic and has since founded the supplement brand

KaraMD. "Eating fresh fruits and vegetables can help with natural energy, improved digestion, reduced disease risk, strengthened cardiovascular health, and more."

But there are plenty of caveats that complicate the issue. We asked experts for their feedback on juicing for weight loss. And although some were cautiously optimistic, others flat-out wouldn't recommend juicing for weight loss. Ahead, here's what the pros have to say.

What is juicing?

Juicing is the practice of extracting juice from fruits and vegetables to make a beverage. This process leaves the fiber behind in the machine (compared with blending up a smoothie, which combines the whole production into the drink). You may choose to do this process at home or to buy pre-made juices.

"Juicing can be used as a supplement to boost nutritional status or as part of a juicing fast," explains Dr. BreAnna Guan, a licensed naturopathic physician specializing in women's hormone health.

Dr. Kien Vuu, M.D., concierge doctor and assistant professor of health sciences at UCLA, says that the removal of the fiber through the juicing process is a major drawback. "The major disadvantage to juicing is losing the healthy fiber content of the fruit or vegetable through the process," he says. "Fiber is important for lowering cholesterol, promoting heart health, regulating blood sugar, and helping feed your gut microbes."

Is juicing good for weight loss?

Experts offer a range of opinions on whether juicing is good for weight loss; typically these opinions range from "under some circumstances" to "no."

Two factors may make it difficult for people to lose weight efficiently, Dr. Kara explains. The first is eating excess calories. And the second is "not getting enough nutrients that the body needs to perform key processes such as metabolizing food," he says.

Given these two factors, juicing can be beneficial for weight loss because it may help replace or supplement what might otherwise be a higher-calorie meal during the day. Further, "nutrient benefits from fresh fruits and vegetables may help promote feelings of fullness for longer and these nutrients provide the body with the fuel it needs to thrive." But, the doctor warns, it's important to be careful when it comes to how juicing is used for weight loss.

"In recent years, juicing or juice 'cleanses' have been misrepresented as easy detoxes or ways to lose weight rapidly," Dr. Kara says. "However, not only is this oftentimes an unsustainable lifestyle in which the weight is gained back at a later date when the juicing is over but replacing most or all of your quality meals with strictly juicing can lead to calorie deficits that may hinder weight loss."

Dr. Vuu is even less optimistic about juicing for weight loss. "I do not consider juicing a viable weight-loss solution," he says plainly. "This form of calorie restriction generally slows down metabolism and [although it] could potentially offer a little bit of weight loss initially, is not a viable long-term option — it may lead to weight gain after the juicing." (Instead, Dr. Vuu recommends intermittent fasting combined with good sleep, exercise, and stress management for weight loss.) It is Dr. Guan's view too that "juicing may be counterproductive for weight loss, especially when using high-glycemic fruits and vegetables such as beets, carrots, apples, and other fruits." These ingredients raise blood sugar, making the breakdown of stored fats more difficult and contributing to the potential for muscle loss. Stephanie Nelson, MS, RD, and MyFitnessPal's lead nutrition scientist, adds: "Remember that to lose weight, you need to consume fewer calories than you burn, so drinking too much juice might lead to consuming more sugar and overall calories than you intended."

Is juicing healthy?

Our experts generally agreed that juicing is healthier as part of a sound nutrition strategy, compared with juicing exclusively for a while. Instead of meal replacement, our experts say juicing can have health benefits when it supplements—not replaces—your existing healthy diet and lifestyle. Dr. Kara says, "using juicing to replace quality meals can lead to extreme calorie deficits while on the other hand supplementing one meal a day, breakfast for example, with juicing can be an easy and convenient way to benefit from the quality nutrients fresh fruits and vegetables have to offer." Ultimately, juicing shouldn't be considered the end-all-be-all of weight loss and health strategies. Rather, it may be one healthy part of an overall strategic approach. "Juicing is best when it is used to complement your already existing health routine; it should not replace making healthy decisions," Dr. Kara says, "If you are keeping up with eating quality meals, engaging in regular physical exercise and stress reduction, and practicing other healthy habits, then juicing can make a great addition to your routine."

Nelson agrees. "My take-home advice is, if you like juice, you can have some as a part of your weight loss regimen," she says. "But make sure you're also getting whole fruits and vegetables because they have some benefits that juice does not."

What's the healthiest way to juice?
Not all juice is created equal for health. "The best juice is that which comes from fresh and organic fruits and vegetables," Dr. Kara explains. "Juices that are pre-made or that use fruits and vegetables that are loaded with preservatives can lead to more issues when it comes to weight as well as one's overall health."

Further, Dr. Kara suggests, the process and type of device used to make the juice also makes a difference. When you include juice and pulp, you get more nutrients that may play an important role in weight loss.

Dr. Guan recommends her clients utilize green juices as a way to support hydration and optimal energy levels, especially during the summer months when dehydration is more of an issue. "Green juices are a great way to supply needed electrolytes that can help improve athletic performance and endurance," she says. "Low-glycemic juicing such as celery, cabbage, kale, and spinach will not raise blood sugar and will be more supportive of weight loss."

Who should avoid juicing?

Dr. Guann advises that juicing can be dangerous for those with eating disorders. Those who are insulin resistant or diabetic should also avoid juicing as it causes much higher spikes in blood sugar when compared to eating the actual fiber-rich fruit or vegetable, Dr. Vuu explains. He adds this caveat: "Before making any major changes

to your lifestyle or diet, it is always best to consult a medical professional."
keto diet side effects, food, dish, cuisine, animal fat, roast beef, meat, ingredient, charcuterie, flesh, veal.

Chapter 6

*Dreamy green juice

You know what they say... an apple a day keeps the doctor away (or in this case, ½ an apple). This simple recipe is packed with green products to help you get your daily dose of fruit + veg, hydrate you, and keep you fuller – for longer. Green Dream Ingredients | Beast Health Recipes Green Dream is a Nutrition Blend – our take on a traditional smoothie – just with more fruits & vegetables optimized with nutrients that boost our immune systems.

To blend, add all ingredients to the Blending Vessel in the order listed. Simply hold down the button for >1 second to initiate the one-minute timed blending cycle.

What Does Green Juice Do to Your Body? Best Seven Reasons

We have heard about the merit of adding leafy greens to your diet, and indeed, they are worthy of praise for all the right reasons. Green juice is the hero of juices. This simple beverage condenses a handful of green veggies and superfoods into a single drink that is stacked with nutrients.

Key Takeaways

Green juice is an extremely rich source of healthy fibers, vitamins, minerals, antioxidants, phytonutrients

Support Your Immune System (thanks to vitamins A & C). Pop into your nearest Pure Green juice bar franchise for your daily dose of delicious, healthy, organic, and cold-pressed green juice

In recent years, green juice and juice bar franchises have gained solid support in wellness circles. Celebrities are drinking them, and wellness juice bloggers praise them. The convenience of getting your daily dose of nutrients appeals to many, and there is no easier way to get this many nutrients in a single serving.

Green juice

Green juice is an extremely rich source of healthy fibers, vitamins, minerals, antioxidants, phytonutrients... the list goes on. It also contains active plant enzymes that your body needs. But what exactly does it do to your body? Read on to find out why you should incorporate more green juice into your diet.

Help Boost the Metabolism of Energy (thanks to vitamin C). What do you do when you are feeling tired and lethargic? Do you reach for a pick-me-up like coffee or an energy drink? Caffeine is fine in moderation, but it only injects a temporary boost – it doesn't tackle the reasons why you are fatigued.

The biology behind your lack of energy is really quite simple; if your body is deprived of nutrients, it doesn't function optimally.

Enter green juices, especially those high in vitamin C, to provide an almost instant energy boost. Unlike stimulants, the release is also gradual, so there is no risk of a crash later during the day.

Drinking green juices on an empty stomach is an excellent source of clean energy delivered directly to your bloodstream.

Support Your Immune System (thanks to vitamins A & C). Our immune systems are much like a car's engine – you will get out what you put in. If you don't replenish your nutrients regularly, things begin to shut down and fail. Zinc and vitamin C deficiencies, for instance, will make you increasingly susceptible to illnesses.

Your leafy greens like broccoli, kale, and spinach are excellent sources of vitamin A and water-soluble vitamin C for easy absorption.

Vitamin C especially is critical to boosting your immunity while dually serving as a potent antioxidant that prevents damage to cells. A regular shot of green juice is the perfect way to replenish everything your immune system needs to keep you healthy.

Contribute to the Health of the Skin (thanks to vitamin A) We have trillions and trillions of cells that will only get clearer and healthier with the right balance of nutrients. Of course, a nutrient-dense diet doesn't just keep your body healthy on the inside, but you will see a visible improvement in your appearance as well. Green juice is one of the quickest and most effective ways to get glowing skin. If you are experiencing dry, dull skin, juice your way to a more youthful appearance.

Green juice will help your skin stay hydrated, while the abundance of vitamin C helps your skin stay firm and radiant. The vitamin K in leafy greens, on the other hand, helps reduce stress, which has a knock-on effect on your appearance. Both the upper and lower layers of your dermis also need vitamin A to produce collagen and prevent sun damage.

Reduces Inflammation

Inflammation is your body's way of telling you that something is wrong. Our bodies work on the Goldilocks principle – our pH levels can be too acidic, too alkaline, or just right. The perfect pH balance falls between 7.35 and 7.45 on the scale.

Generally, our bodies are equipped to self-regulate the pH balance to the ideal range, but modern diets and the consumption of alcohol can throw this out of whack.

Buffering minerals are then pulled from other areas that the body needs to maintain pH levels, leaving you with deficiencies. With a diet that is too acidic, for instance, calcium and magnesium are taken from the bones to balance the score.

Incorporating green veggies not only helps to balance your pH levels but also to reduce painful inflammation internally and externally. The easiest way to get your daily dose is through a glass of green juice. Your body will feel and perform better overall.

Improved Digestion

It is not known to many people, but your gut biome is the starting point of your health. It can literally affect your mood and your happiness. Drinking green juice will support gut health through probiotics. These tiny microorganisms found in the juice will support the growth of healthy bacteria in the digestive tract.

Aids in Weight Loss

Losing weight, burning more energy, and improving digestion go hand in hand. Because green juice is so low in empty calories and nutrient-dense, they are a great way to replace a morning or afternoon snack.

You will kick start your metabolism, have more energy to exercise and feel fuller. It is worth a mention that your green juice can supplement your daily veggie intake, but it is not really a full meal replacement.

Detoxifies

No matter how health-conscious or how careful we are, our bodies are put through the wringer every day by being exposed to toxins. You can't escape it – we are exposed to toxins in the air we breathe. As we have mentioned, free radicals lead to various diseases and speed up the aging process.

Not only is green juice packed with antioxidants that combat these free radicals, but it also supports your liver in excreting the harmful toxins that strain your organs.

Cruciferous veggies like the ones found in quality green drinks can improve what is called phase II detoxification of the liver, so your body will expel toxins rapidly.

A Pep in Your Step with Pure Green Juice

Pop into your nearest Pure Green juice bar franchise for your daily dose of delicious, healthy, organic, and cold-pressed green juice. They do not sneak in flavorings or added sugars, so you are guaranteed to get the best for your body. Not living near a Pure Green juice bar franchise? Don't stress – they deliver right to your door! You can choose between three yummy green juice options and one booster shot;

All three juices have kale, spinach, cucumber, celery, zucchini, and romaine as base juice.

Pure Green Alg is mixed with apple, lemon, and ginger for extra goodness and flavor. Pure Green Apple boasts a dash of appley sweetness, and Pure Green LG packs a zesty punch with lemon and ginger. Our Green Boost shot contains kale, spinach, apple, cucumber, mint, and spirulina.

www.ingramcontent.com/pod-product-compliance
Lightning Source LLC
Chambersburg PA
CBHW071028260726
48662CB00024B/2157